# NUTRITION
## in the
# CHEMO CHAIR

## From an Oncology Dietitian's Perspective

Jennifer Fitzgibbon, MS, RDN, CSO, CDN

To order additional copies of this book, contact:
Xlibris
1-888-795-4274
www.Xlibris.com
Orders@Xlibris.com

ISBN:    Softcover        978-1-7960-8588-4
         EBook            978-1-7960-8587-7

Print information available on the last page

Rev. date: 01/29/2020

# CONTENTS

Hearing the words, *"you have cancer"* for the first time is life altering. New thoughts, fears, struggles, and possibly new responsibilities are often the primary focus at this time. Nutrition is often a new thought for many, as there are many strong associations with healthy eating, weight, activity, and how these things have influence on cancer.

Learning about your treatment options is a discussion at this time. For many, chemotherapy is part of the plan.

## WHAT IS CHEMOTHERAPY?

Chemotherapy is the use of anti-cancer drugs to treat cancer. It can stop the growth of a tumor and kill cancer cells that have spread to other parts of the body. Chemotherapy may also be used to reduce the risk of cancer returning (recurrence), and to shrink the size of a tumor to reduce cancer-related symptoms.

## WHEN IS IT CHEMOTHERAPY GIVEN?

Chemotherapy may be given after surgery (called *adjuvant chemotherapy*) or before surgery (known as *neoadjuvant chemotherapy*). Chemotherapy usually starts within 4 to 12 weeks after surgery (if part of you treatment), or upon diagnosis. It is commonly given in cycles. The length of the cycle will depend on the type of drugs used. The length of the treatment period will vary, but it may last from 3 to 6 months, sometimes in addition to radiation therapy.

## HOW IS CHEMOTHERAPY GIVEN?

Anti-cancer drugs are taken by mouth or injected into the muscle or fat tissue below the skin; but most are injected into a vein. Treatments can be given at home, at the doctor's office or in the hospital — depending on the type of chemotherapy.

Several topics exist regarding weight and cancer including with how well you tolerate and respond to treatments such as chemotherapy. There is also evidence in regards to weight and the growth of new or pre-existing cancer cells once they have stopped or slowed by treatment.

# OBESITY

## Position Statement

Rates of obesity have increased significantly over the last three decades in the United States and globally. (1) In addition to contributing to heart disease and diabetes, obesity is a major unrecognized risk factor for cancer. (1) Research shows that the time after a cancer diagnosis can serve as a teachable moment to motivate individuals to adopt risk-reducing behaviors. (1) For this reason, the oncology care team—the providers with whom a patient has the closest relationships in the critical period after a cancer diagnosis—is in a unique position to help patients lose weight and make other healthy lifestyle changes. (1) The American Society of Clinical Oncology is committed to reducing the impact of obesity on cancer and has established a multipronged initiative to accomplish this goal by 1) increasing education and awareness of the evidence linking obesity and cancer; 2) providing tools and resources to help oncology providers address obesity with their patients; 3) building and fostering a robust research agenda to better understand the pathophysiology of energy balance alterations, evaluate the impact of behavior change on cancer outcomes, and determine the best methods to help cancer survivors make effective and useful changes in lifestyle behaviors; and 4) advocating for policy and systems change to address societal factors contributing to obesity and improve access to weight management services for patients with cancer. (1)

## Economic Burden of Obesity and Cancer

A projection of the future health and economic burden of obesity in 2030 estimated that continuation of existing trends in obesity will lead to about 500,000 additional cases of cancer in the United States by 2030. This analysis also found that if every adult reduced their BMI by 1 percent, which would be equivalent to a weight loss of roughly 1 kg (or 2.2 lbs) for an adult of average weight, this would prevent the increase in the number of cancer cases and actually result in the *avoidance* of about 100,000 new cases of cancer. (2)

## Hormonal Associations with Obesity and Cancer

Several possible mechanisms have been suggested to explain the association of obesity with increased risk of certain cancers:

- o Fat tissue produces excess amounts of a hormone known as estrogen. Elevated estrogen levels have been associated with the risk of breast, endometrial, and some other cancers.(3)
- o Obese people often have increased levels of insulin and *insulin-like growth factor-1 (IGF-1)* in their blood (a condition known as hyperinsulinemia or insulin resistance), which may promote the development of certain tumors.(3)
- o Fat cells produce hormones, called adipokines that may stimulate or inhibit cell growth. For example, a hormone known as leptin, which is more abundant in obese people, seems to promote cell growth, whereas, another hormone known as adiponectin, which is less abundant in obese people, and may slow tumor growth. (3)
- o Obese people often have chronic low-level, or "subacute," inflammation, which has been associated with increased cancer risk.(3)

# WEIGHT LOSS OR MALNUTRITION

All patients with cancer should be considered at risk for inadequate calorie and nutrient intake. (4) It is estimated that malnutrition affects up to 80% of patients with certain cancers, including cancer of the head and neck, gastrointestinal tract cancer, and pancreatic cancer. (4) Malnutrition is considered the cause of 20–40% of all cancer-related deaths. (4)

## Why do People Lose Weight With Cancer?

### "The Rut"

Cancer can cause chemical changes that make it very difficult for you to gain weight, sometimes even if you are eating a high calorie diet. These chemicals are probably the cause of cachexia or "*the rut*" - the severe weight loss that some people have with advanced cancer.

Chemicals that the cancer produces may make your body work at a faster rate than normal, even when you are resting. In other words, you can have a higher than normal metabolic rate.

The 2006 Cachexia Consensus Conference, established cachexia as "a complex metabolic syndrome associated with underlying illness and characterized by loss of muscle with or without loss of fat mass (6). Cancer-induced cachexia (CIC) is experienced by up to 80% of patients with advanced stage cancer, particularly those with gastrointestinal, pancreatic, thoracic and head and neck malignancies. CIC has been implicated in up to 20% of cancer-related deaths. (7, 8)

A cancer can produce chemicals that affect the way your normal cells work. Some of these chemicals are called *cytokines*. These are made normally by your immune system and released into your body when you get an infection. Cytokines help your body fight infection but they are also responsible for how you feel when you get an infection. High cytokine levels make you feel as if you have a cold or flu.

A cancer can make cytokines in larger than normal amounts. These can cause weight loss and muscle wasting by making your body break down fat and protein faster than normal. They may also affect the center in the brain that controls hunger.

Another chemical cancers can produce is *'proteolysis-inducing factor'* (PIF) (45). It seems to have something to do with weight loss and muscle wasting in people with cancer. PIF is only found in the blood and urine of people with cancer who are losing weight. You don't find it in people who don't have cancer or in people who do have cancer, but are not losing weight.

During this biological cascade of events "the rut" creates a disconnection of "body-telling-brain" you are hungry or even thirsty. It is this innate chemical loss that people have a very difficult time with, even if there is no sense of nausea, there is no sense of want or desire for food and many times the subconscious oral-saliva- swallow is diminished or disappears making it extremely difficult to functionally eat or even drink.

## Inflammation due to cancer

Some types of cancer make the tissue around them become inflamed. The inflammation makes your body release more cytokines into your bloodstream so the levels of these chemicals will be even higher. Because of this theory, studies are done using anti-inflammatory drugs to treat cachexia.

## Omega-3 fat

Omega-3 fats can regulate inflammatory processes and responses. Researchers recently investigated omega-3s and other fats (such as omega-6 fats and alpha linolenic acid) to see if their consumption was associated with a reduction in mortality due to inflammatory diseases. (9)

For cancer patients, consuming a diet high in omega-3 fats could help them maintain and even regain lost muscle mass. Most patients who took a daily supplement for 10 weeks either maintained or gained muscle mass. Patients who didn't take anything either maintained or lost muscle mass. (10)

## Nutritional Tips to Lower Your Inflammatory Process

Lifestyle changes such as those noted below are very effective at reducing chronic inflammation in your body:

- **Focus on eating a healthy diet.** This includes avoiding pro-inflammatory foods like Trans fats, fried foods, sugar, fructose and grains, foods cooked at high temperatures and oxidized cholesterol (cholesterol that has gone rancid, such as that from overcooked, scrambled eggs).
- **Get plenty of high quality omega-3 fats.** There are two major types of omega-3 fatty acids in our diets: One type is alpha-linolenic acid (ALA), which is found in some vegetable oils, such as soybean, rapeseed (canola), and flaxseed, and in walnuts. ALA is also found in some green vegetables, such as Brussel sprouts, kale, spinach, and salad greens. The other type, eicosapentanoic acid (EPA) and docosahexanoic acid (DHA), is found in fatty fish. The body partially converts ALA to EPA and DHA.
It is unclear whether vegetable or fish omega-3 fatty acids are equally beneficial, although both seem to be beneficial. Unfortunately, most Americans do not get enough of either type. For good health, you should aim to get at least one rich source of omega-3 fatty acids in your diet every day. This could be through a serving of fatty fish (such as wild-caught salmon), a tablespoon of canola or soybean oil in salad dressing or in cooking, or a handful of walnuts or ground flaxseed mixed into your morning oatmeal.
- **Optimize your insulin levels.** If your fasting insulin level is not lower than three, consider limiting your intake of grains and sugars until you optimize your insulin level.
- **Optimize your vitamin D levels.** Most people are not aware that vitamin D deficiency is associated with inflammation, so you will want to be sure your levels are in the healthy range by eating foods high in vitamin D and taking a high-quality vitamin D3 supplement.
- **Exercise regularly.** Exercise is a great way to lower inflammation without any of the side effects associated with medications. The American Institute of Cancer Research recommends 30 minutes of activity daily.
- **Make sure your waist size is normal.** If you're a woman with a waist measurement of over 35 inches or a man with a waist of over 40 inches, you probably have high inflammation and should take steps to lose weight.

## Why do Some People Lose Weight During Chemo?

People receiving chemotherapy lose weight because chemotherapy can damage healthy cells in the lining of the digestive system. Your whole digestive system can be affected. The digestive system extends from the mouth to the anus and includes the salivary glands, stomach, intestines, and rectum. Chemotherapy can affect these areas and cause nausea, vomiting, diarrhea, constipation, fatigue, pain, and mouth sores.

Some digestive system side effects, such as vomiting, may become severe enough to delay your chemotherapy treatment. Or your medical team may opt to reduce your dose of chemotherapy to help lessen the symptoms of digestive side effects. Receiving your planned dose of chemo may help you get the most out of your treatment. That's why it's important to speak with your medical team about doing all that you can to avoid having to reduce or delay your chemo treatment.

## Nausea and Vomiting

Weight loss occurs because many people on chemotherapy may experience nausea and vomiting. Many chemo drugs cause the release of a substance called serotonin and other chemicals. This release can be a signal that activates the "*vomiting center*" in your brain.

The nausea and vomiting caused by chemo can be:

- *Acute*: Occurs within minutes to the first few hours after chemotherapy administration
- *Delayed*: Occurs 24 hours or more after chemotherapy
- *Anticipatory:* Occurs as a conditioned response, meaning it happens in response to stimulus that has caused nausea or vomiting in the past, such as the sight or smells of the treatment room.

Certain chemotherapy medicines are more likely than others to cause nausea and vomiting. Chemo drugs are classified as minimal, low, moderate, or high in terms of the chance they will cause vomiting. If the chemotherapy prescribed for you is associated with a moderate to high probability of nausea and vomiting, your medical team will likely recommend appropriate support medicines to control the chemo side effects. Discuss your chemo regimen with your medical team. Ask what the likelihood is that you will experience nausea and vomiting as a result of your treatment.

## What Can Be Done to Manage Nausea and Vomiting?

Medicines for controlling nausea and vomiting are called antiemetic's. Some of these drugs block the signal in the brain and gut that causes nausea and vomiting. You may have you to try more than one antiemetic medication before finding the prescription that works best for you.

There are also several things you can do at home to help prevent or control nausea and vomiting:

- Eat 5 to 6 smaller meals, rather than 3 large meals, throughout the day.
- Eat foods that are easy to digest. Foods that are not as likely to upset your stomach include dry cereal, plain crackers, rice, and toast. (See examples included adapted from the Fact Sheets on Managing Nausea and vomiting from the National Cancer Institute)
- Try ginger, mint, and tea.
- Be sure to keep properly hydrated, dehydration may contribute to nausea.
- Avoid onions, garlic, coffee, and other strong-smelling foods. Avoid being around food as it is being cooked.
- Wait at least 1 hour after your chemo before eating or drinking anything.
- Consume foods and drinks at room temperature or cool.
- If you feel the urge to vomit, try slow, deep breathing.
- You may be able to distract yourself by reading, watching television, or doing a relaxing hobby.

- Ask your medical team about medicine for controlling nausea and vomiting during and after chemotherapy. Do not wait until after you feel nauseas to take the medicine, try and take the medicine pre-mealtime if you have ongoing nausea.

| <u>Soups</u> | <u>Drinks</u> | <u>Main meals and snacks</u> | <u>Fruits and sweets</u> |
|---|---|---|---|
| Clear broth, such as chicken, beef, and vegetable | Clear soda, such as ginger ale Cranberry or grape juice Oral rehydration drinks, such as Pedialyte® | Chicken—broiled or baked without the skin | Bananas |
| | | Cream of wheat or rice cereal | Canned fruit such as applesauce, peaches, and pears |
| | | Crackers or pretzels | Gelatin (Jell-O®) |
| | Tea | Oatmeal | Popsicles and sherbet |
| | Water | Pasta or noodles | Yogurt (plain or vanilla |
| | | Potatoes—boiled/ without the skin | |
| | | White rice / White toast | |

## Medications that improve appetite

Sometimes medications, called appetite stimulants, are used for people with poor appetite and weight loss. They can help some people but not everyone. The most commonly used appetite stimulants are:

- Megesterol acetate
- Medroxyprogesterone acetate
- Marinol (Cannabis)

A recent review of research showed that Megesterol acetate increases appetite and weight gain, but is no more effective than steroids. As both types of drugs have side effects, more research is needed to find out how much Megesterol acetate improves overall quality of life. (4)

Other appetite stimulants being tested include cannabinoids. These drugs are made from the cannabis plant, also known as marijuana. Some studies have found that smoking cannabis or eating it can help to control sickness and pain and increase appetite. But some research failed to show that cannabinoids improved appetite or quality of life. Neither does it seem to help people put on weight.

## Constipation

Constipation is difficulty passing stool. It can also refer to a decrease in the normal frequency of bowel movements. It may be accompanied by gas, pain, or pressure in the abdomen which can create problems eating causing weight loss.

Constipation is a chemo side effect that can often be managed by diet or by medication.

Your medical team will want to make sure that you are having regular bowel movements during chemo. Chronic constipation can lead to something called stool impaction. This occurs when the stool gets stuck and cannot pass through the colon or rectum. Impaction can be a very serious complication of constipation.

### Causes of Constipation

Constipation can have a number of causes, including:

- Chemotherapy drugs
- Drugs given to reduce pain
- Decreased physical activity
- Not eating enough foods with fiber
- Not drinking enough water or other fluids

### Symptoms

Symptoms of constipation include:

- Fewer bowel movements than what is normal for you
- Hard, difficult-to-pass bowel movements
- Cramping or stomach-ache
- Flatulence (gas)

### Prevention Tips

It is easier to prevent constipation with lifestyle changes than to treat it once it happens. Here are some tips:

*Three important factors for normal bowel motility: Fluids plus Fiber plus Activity*

- Drink plenty of water. Fluids keep the stool soft.
- Eat foods high in fiber; these include fruit, vegetables, and nuts, try for 25-35 grams of fiber daily, if you bowel can tolerate.
- If your doctor approves, exercise daily. Exercise helps stimulate digestion and prevent constipation. Even moderate activity, such as walking, will help.

Keep track of your bowel movement schedule so you can learn which lifestyle measures work best for you. If you miss a bowel movement, try increasing your fluid intake or adjusting your diet. Call your doctor if your bowels have not moved in 2 days; your doctor may choose to prescribe a laxative or other medication.

## Management

If you have tried the above lifestyle changes and still experience constipation, your doctor may prescribe laxatives. Laxatives are available in many forms, including tablets, gum, powder, granules, or as a liquid.

Let your care team know if you have signs or symptoms of constipation. Ask your healthcare provider which type of laxative or stool softener will work best for you. As with all treatments, speak with your doctor and health care team about the risks and benefits of treatments for constipation.

# Diarrhea

Chemotherapy can damage the cells in your mouth, and all along the lining of the intestine, which, in turn, can cause diarrhea (watery or loose stools). You should contact your medical team if you have diarrhea that lasts for more than 24 hours, and/or if you have pain and cramping that accompany the diarrhea. It is important that you replace the water and nutrients you have lost.

Your physician may prescribe a medication to control your symptoms, and/or, if symptoms persist, you may need fluid replacement intravenously (IV). It is possible to replace these fluids intravenously on an outpatient basis. When you are having chemotherapy, you should not take any over-the-counter medications for diarrhea without first consulting your medical team.

## Nutritional Recommendations for Diarrhea

If you have diarrhea, consider foods such as the following:

- rice, noodles, and potatoes
- farina and cream of wheat
- eggs (cooked until the whites are solid, avoid frying in fat)
- smooth peanut butter
- white bread
- peeled fruits, and well-cooked vegetables
- skinned chicken or turkey, lean beef, and fish (broiled or baked, not fried)

With diarrhea, try to avoid the following types of foods:

- fatty and fried foods
- raw vegetables

- fruit seeds, skins, and stringy fibers
- vegetables high in fiber such as broccoli, corn, dried beans, cabbage, peas, and cauliflower
- Some people need to avoid milk and dairy products when they have diarrhea. This is because they may not tolerate the lactose contained in these products.

In addition, consider the following information provided by the National Cancer Institute (NCI) as ways to reduce the severity of your symptoms:

- Be sure to replace all fluids that you have lost by drinking plenty of water and other fluid, such as clear broth, electrolytes beverages (try sugarless versions), plain coconut water, or natural ginger ale. If you choose a carbonated beverage, let it sit for a while until it loses its carbonation.
- Eat small meals throughout the day instead of three large meals.
- Diarrhea can cause you to lose potassium. Unless your doctor has told you otherwise, eat potassium-rich foods such as bananas, oranges, potatoes, and diluted peach and apricot nectars.
- Ask your medical team if it is advisable to temporarily switch to a clear liquid diet to give your bowels time to rest. However, this kind of diet does not provide all of the nutrients you will need and should not be followed for more than three to five days.

  - Choose foods that are low in fiber, such as the following:

    - white bread
    - white rice or noodles
    - creamed cereals
    - ripe bananas
    - canned (packed in water)or cooked fruit without skins
    - yogurt (if able to tolerate) without seeds
    - eggs
    - mashed or baked potatoes without the skin
    - pureed vegetables, chicken, or turkey without the skin
    - fish
    - Avoid high-fiber foods that may cause diarrhea and cramping. These include whole grain breads and cereals, raw vegetables, beans, nuts, seeds, popcorn, and fresh and dried fruit. Other foods that may cause cramping and diarrhea include coffee, tea with caffeine, alcohol, sweets, and fried, greasy, or highly spiced foods.
    - Avoid milk and milk products*, including ice cream, as diary may aggravate your symptoms.
    - *You can replace milk products with alternatives such as almond milk, soy milk, or coconut milk. Or you can try lactaid milk or lactaid tablets to help with digestion.

## Fatigue

Fatigue, (a persistent sense of tiredness or exhaustion) is the most common symptom reported by patients receiving chemotherapy. This is caused by the rapid destruction of cells in the body, along with the need to rebuild.

Cancer-related fatigue is a persistent feeling of physical, emotional, or mental tiredness or exhaustion related to cancer and/or its treatment. This type of fatigue is different than other types of fatigue, such as when a healthy person does not get enough rest, because it interferes with a person's usual functioning, does not reflect their level of activity, and does not improve with rest. Most people receiving cancer treatment experience fatigue, usually within a few days of chemotherapy, and some cancer survivors have fatigue that lasts for months and sometimes years after finishing treatment.

## How Fatigue Affects Your Nutritional Status:

Fatigue often negatively affects the overall physical, psychological, social, and economic well-being of a person with cancer. For some, it is slightly bothersome, while for others the experience can be overwhelming. Fatigue may influence you're:

- Daily activities; including cooking, food shopping, general eating activities
- Hobbies and other enjoyable activities
- Social relationships
- Mood and emotions
- Job performance
- Feeling of well-being and sense of joy
- Attitude toward the future
- Ability to undergo treatment

## Pain

Chemotherapy can cause pain for some people, including headaches, muscle pain, stomach pain, and pain from nerve damage, such as burning, numbness, or shooting pains (most often in the fingers and toes). Pain usually decreases over time, but some people may have symptoms for months or years after chemotherapy has finished due to permanent damage to the nerves.

## Mouth Sores

Mucositis (also known as stomatitis) is the swelling, irritation, and ulceration of the cells that line the digestive tract. These cells reproduce rapidly and have a shorter life span than other cells in the body. Because chemotherapy agents do not differentiate between healthy cells and cancer cells, they can quickly destroy digestive tract cells, breaking down the protective lining and leaving them inflamed, irritated, and swollen. Mucositis can occur anywhere along the digestive tract from the mouth to the anus, and can be aggravated by nausea and vomiting.

## What are the Symptoms of Mucositis?

- redness, dryness, or swelling of the mouth
- burning or discomfort when eating or drinking
- open sores in the mouth and throat, abdominal cramps, or tenderness
- rectal redness or ulcers

## Nutritional Management and Goals

Ensure adequate hydration and maintain or improve overall nutritional status by eating non-irritating, nutrient dense foods and fluids.

> However, patients with severe **mucositis** of the mouth and throat and **esophagitis** may find it too painful and difficult to eat, and a more aggressive nutritional support is needed (Grade 4 toxicity).

The National Cancer Institute created originally the Common Toxicity Criteria (CTC) to aid in the recognition and grading severity of adverse effects caused by chemotherapy treatments.

### NCI-CTCAE Grading Scale

| Grade | Description |
|---|---|
| Grade 0 (none) | None |
| Grade 1 (mild) | Painless ulcers, erythema, or mild soreness in the absence of lesions |
| Grade 2 (moderate) | Painful erythema, edema, or ulcers but eating or swallowing possible |
| Grade 3 (severe) | Painful erythema, edema, or ulcers requiring IV hydration |
| Grade 4 (life-threatening) | Severe ulceration or requiring parenteral or enteral nutritional support or prophylactic intubation |
| Grade 5 (death) | Death related to toxicity |

Encourage good oral hygiene practices to promote comfort, enhance taste and stimulate appetite. A basic regime of oral care, including gentle teeth brushing, flossing and rinsing is essential to minimize the risk of developing oral complications.

Encourage the use of bicarbonate rinses (½ tsp. baking soda dissolved in 2 cups of water), before and after meals.

Discourage intake of known irritants such as:

- Tart or acidic foods or fluids
- Spicy, salty or very sweet foods or fluids
- Dry or rough foods
- Tobacco, alcohol, alcohol-based mouth washes, alcohol-based liquid
- Vitamins
- Reinforce the use of pain medications as prescribed by physician
- Encourage adequate fluid intake. Well-tolerated fluids include warm or cool milk based beverages, non-acidic fruit drinks- (diluted if necessary), "flat "carbonated beverages, cream soups, blended or calorie and/or protein fortified broth based soups.
- Alter the consistency and temperature of foods to suit individual tolerances (for example cool or lukewarm temperature, soft solids, mashed solids, pureed solids, baby foods, thick or thin liquids).
- Recommend dunking or moistening dry foods in liquid.
- Recommend small, frequent energy and protein dense meals or snacks.
- Ensure vitamin and mineral needs are met if nutrition modifications are to be long term.

### *If nutrient supplementation is necessary, suggest:*

- Crushing a multivitamin/mineral tablet and taking it with liquid
- Using a blender to crush the tablet when making a blenderized drink/meal
- A low alcohol liquid vitamin supplement (ask pharmacist for examples)
- A children's chewable multivitamin/mineral supplement

## Nutritional Supplements to Help With Mucositis

### Glutamine

Glutamine has been shown to reduce the degree of mucositis through: anti-inflammatory mechanisms, inhibition of bacterial toxins increased tissue healing and increased fibroblast and collagen synthesis.

Is Glutamine Safe To Give To Patients With Cancer?

Although known to be controversial, under certain circumstances cancer cells use glutamine for energy even more voraciously than glucose. Tumors differ according to their need for glutamine, (31) and, no human study, have ever shown that glutamine increased tumor growth rates or decreased the efficacy of other cancer. (32) Over the last 20 years, researchers have demonstrated the tolerance, safety and effects of glutamine (oral and IV) in patients undergoing chemotherapy and/or radiation therapy (32). In each of these studies, researchers have reported that glutamine supplementation in cancer patients improves their metabolism and clinical situation without increasing tumor growth (32).

Help to Prevent Mucositis

You can buy glutamine (*usually in the form of L-glutamine*), in powder, capsule, tablet, or liquid form. Examples are, *Designs for Health L-glutamine Powder or Nestle Glutasolve.*

Some recommendations use the powder form of L-glutamine, and mixing it in with cold or room temperature liquids (water or juice.) (31) It should not be added to hot beverages because heat destroys glutamine. Glutamine therapy works best if started at the time of beginning chemotherapy. It will be less effective if you start this after already showing signs or symptoms of mucositis.

- DOSE: Mix 10 grams of powdered glutamine in a small glass (6-8 ounces) of water or non-acidic juice. Swish and gargle for 30-60 seconds and swallow. You can continue to do this until the 6-8 ounces are gone. Repeat every 8 hours (schedule: morning, mid-day, evening)
- Start this regimen on the first day of chemotherapy and continue for 14 days after the last dose of chemotherapy in patients who do not develop oral mucositis or until 5 days after resolution of oral mucositis for patients who experienced oral mucositis. (33)

*Other recommendations:*

  o Refrain from eating or drinking for 30 minutes after dosing.
  o Adhere to good oral hygiene practices and gently brushed their teeth twice daily, 30 minutes or more after using glutamine, using a soft toothbrush and fluoride toothpaste.
  o Daily flossing and an alcohol-free fluoride rinse is recommended.

- Another suggestion involves swallowing the following dose (verses swish and spit) and is based on a study (31) that showed a significant reduction in oral mucositis among patients using oral glutamine.

  o These investigators used a proprietary glutamine suspension *(Saforis, MGI Pharma, Inc., Bloomington, MN),* which was administered at a dose of:
    - 2.5 grams per 5 mL 3 times per day for a total daily dose of 7.5 g.
    - This product reportedly is able to be better absorbed into the oral mucosa than standard glutamine.

For help to prevent mucositis of the <u>throat and esophagus</u> *(esophagitis)* from radiation and chemotherapy:

- *DOSE: Mix 10 grams of powdered glutamine in a small glass (6-8 ounces) of water or juice. Drink (swallow). Repeat every 8 hours (schedule: morning, mid-day, evening)*
- *Start this regimen 1 week before radiation therapy and continue for 2 weeks after completion of radiation therapy. (31)*

## Honey

One of the most effective therapies to help reduce the severity and pain of mucositis comes from pure natural honey. The viscous nature of honey makes it a great protective barrier that coats the delicate mucous membranes of the mouth and throat. Organic Manuka Honey 5ml / 4 times a day / held in mouth for 30 seconds /then swallowed has been shown to help with mucositis. It is inexpensive and has no side effects. Honey also has natural bactericidal properties that help protect against increased colonization by bacterial and fungal organisms. (34, 35)

Examples: *"Wedderspoon Premium Raw Manuka Honey Active 12+"*

## Aloe Vera

Aloe Vera used as a mouthwash can be effective for mouth sores and mouth ulcers, it's particularly known for its ability to heal burns. Aloe Vera juice can be used, with a little honey to help the taste. Aloe Vera juice can be ordered on-line or found at health food stores.

Aloe Vera gel can also be used. (36)

## Ice Cubes

Sucking on ice chips before, during, or right after the chemotherapy session might minimize the severity of the sores, particularly if 5-FU is the chemotherapy drug being used. (37) Research has also shown that there is a difference in the experiences of the patients while sucking plain ice cubes and flavored ice cubes. As a whole, the results showed that the flavored ice cubes were effective in preventing mucositis and the patients were in favor of the flavored ice cubes. (38)

# Weight Gain During Chemo

Although it is more common to lose weight during cancer treatment, some people gain weight. Slight increases in weight during cancer treatment are generally not problematic. However, significant weight gain may affect a person's health and ability to undergo treatment.

Weight gain is an especially relevant health issue for women with breast cancer because more than half experience weight gain during treatment. Evidence has shown that weight gain during treatment is linked to a poorer prognosis (chance of recovery). Being overweight before treatment begins also increases the risk of serious health conditions, such as high blood pressure, diabetes, and cardiovascular disease.

## Causes

The following cancer treatments may produce symptoms that lead to weight gain:

- **Chemotherapy:** Some chemotherapy causes the body to retain (hold on to) excess fluid in cells and tissues, which is called edema. In addition, chemotherapy often causes people to reduce physical activity, usually because of fatigue; increases hunger, especially for high-fat foods; triggers intense food cravings; and decreases metabolism (the rate that the body uses energy). It may also cause menopause in some women, which decreases their metabolism, increasing the likelihood of weight gain.

- **Steroid medications:** Steroids are medications that are often used for cancer treatment to reduce symptoms of inflammation, such as swelling and pain. For some cancers, they are used as part of the treatment for the cancer itself. A side effect of these medications is an increase in fatty issue, resulting in a large abdomen and fullness in the neck or face. Steroids may also cause wasting (loss of both weight and muscle mass). A noticeable increase in weight usually only occurs when people have been taking steroids continuously for many weeks.
- **Hormone therapy:** Hormone therapy for the treatment of breast, uterine, prostate, and testicular cancers involves medications that decrease the amount of estrogen or progesterone in women and testosterone in men. This can increase body mass from fat, decrease body mass from muscle, and decrease metabolism, resulting in weight gain.

## Managing weight gain

Relieving side effects–€also called *"symptom management, palliative care, or supportive care"* is an important part of cancer care and treatment. Talk with your health care team about any symptoms you experience, including any new symptoms or a change in symptoms.

If weight gain becomes a concern, consult with your medical team or a registered dietitian (RD) before starting a diet or changing eating habits. They can help discover the possible cause of the weight gain and find the best way to manage it. In addition, an RD can provide nutritional guidelines or a customized diet plan.

Consider the following ways to address weight gain through diet and physical activity:

- Eat plenty of fruits, vegetables, and whole grains.
- Limit fat, sugar, salt, and refined flour.
- Drink plenty of water.
- Try to use healthier cooking methods whenever possible, such as steaming instead of frying.
- Evaluate everyday eating habits, and try to identify behavior patterns that lead to overeating and inactivity.
- Find cardiovascular physical activities (such as walking or bicycling) that you enjoy, and do strength building exercises if muscle mass has been lost. However, check with your doctor before beginning a new type of exercise or increasing your amount of physical activity.

## Managing fluid retention-related weight gain

It is important to call your doctor immediately if you experience any of the following signs of fluid retention:

- Skin that feels stiff or leaves small indentations on the skin after pressing on the swollen area
- Swelling of the arms or legs, especially around the ankles and wrists
- Rings, wristwatches, bracelets, or shoes that fit tighter than usual
- Decreased flexibility in the hands, elbows, wrists, fingers, or legs

The following tips can help you manage fluid retention:

- Ask a doctor about prescribing a diuretic medication (medication that increases urination) to rid the body of excess water.
- Lower the amount of salt in your diet.

# CALORIES DURING CHEMOTHERAPY

It is recommended to eat a pattern of small, frequent meals, that is, four to six small meals a day that are high in calories, protein and other nutrients to help promote appetite and adequate overall nutrition for energy level and immune support.

Protein shakes or smoothies are often a helpful way of reaching these goals. The protein powders that are recommended most often include whey or soy protein powder, which can be found at a variety of health food stores and grocery or drug stores.

Canola oil will not change the texture or flavor of the shake. Other tips for boosting total calories without increasing the volume of food include using healthful fats such as olive oil; nut butters (peanut, almond, sunflower seed, etc.); pesto, snacking on nuts/trail mix/granola; and using whole-milk dairy products.

## Why is protein important during chemotherapy?

Protein is very important to keep your body functioning and is also needed for growth and repair. Protein is found in almost all body cells and has many roles such as:

- To form and maintain muscles, tissues, red blood cells, enzymes, and hormones
- To carry many body compounds and medications
- To maintain fluid balance
- To fight infections and strengthen the immune system

In general, your diet will provide enough protein. However, during cancer treatment (such as surgery, radiation therapy and chemotherapy) your protein requirements may increase. It is important to be aware of your protein requirements, food sources of protein and to include these foods at meals and snacks.

## Your protein requirements

To come up with a quick estimate of your protein requirement:

- Take your weight (in pounds) and divide by 2
- The number you get is the approximate number of grams of protein you need daily

For example: If you weigh 180 pounds, 180 ÷ 2 = 90 grams of protein daily

If you are receiving chemotherapy, radiation or surgery you may need more protein. Your dietitian can help you figure out your protein needs during treatment.

## Food sources of protein

Protein is found in both animal and plant foods. Animal sources of protein include meat, poultry, fish, eggs and dairy products. Plant sources of protein include nuts, seeds, tofu and legumes (dried beans, peas and lentils). Grains (cereals, breads and rice) and vegetables contain a little protein. Fruits and fats do not have any protein.

## Protein content of foods

### Food Serving Grams of Protein

- Meat - beef, pork, lamb: 3 oz 21 grams
- Poultry - chicken, turkey 3 oz 21 grams
- Fish 3 oz 21 grams
- Egg or ¼ cup liquid egg 7 grams
- Milk 1 cup 8 grams
- Yogurt 1 cup 8-18 grams
- Cottage or ricotta cheese ½ cup 12 grams
- Hard cheese 1 oz 8 grams
- Dried beans and legumes ½ cup 8 grams
- Tofu ½ cup 14 grams
- Nuts ¼ cup 7 grams
- Peanut butter 2 Tbs 7 grams
- Vegetables ½ cup cooked 2 grams
- Starches -1 sl bread, ½ cup rice
- or pasta, 1 serving cereal 2 grams
- Fruit 0
- Fats 0

### High protein snacks

- Cheese with crackers, vegetables or fruit
- Trail mix (mixture of assorted nuts and dried fruits)
- Granola, energy and breakfast bars
- Cereal and milk
- Yogurt
- Cottage cheese or ricotta cheese with fruit
- Chicken, tuna or egg salad on crackers
- Deviled and hard-boiled eggs
- Hot cocoa (if using instant cocoa replace water with milk)
- Puddings and custards
- A glass of regular, flavored or malted milk
- Nuts
- Peanut butter on crackers
- Hummus (a dip made with garbanzo beans)

### Ways to add protein to food

- Shredded cheese - sprinkle over vegetables, potatoes, noodles, casseroles, soups or salads
- Milk - use in place of water when making soups or cooked cereals

- Hard-cooked eggs - chop and add to salads, vegetables or casseroles
- Left-over meat, chicken or fish - add to soups, salads or omelets
- Nuts and seeds - sprinkle over vegetables, fruits, salads, yogurt, cereal and pasta
- Dried beans - add to salads, pasta or soups

## Calories and protein

To make sure that the protein you eat is used for important body functions you must eat enough calories. If you lose weight, your body will use protein for energy rather than to support important body functions.

## Protein supplements

If you are not eating enough protein you may need to use protein supplements. The most economical and easiest protein supplement is dry skim milk powder. Mix the powder with liquid milk to increase the protein content. Also, add dry milk powder to any creamy foods such as mashed potatoes, casseroles, scrambled eggs and creamed soups. You can also add it to pancake and muffin batter. Use pasteurized egg substitute in shakes and recipes as a protein supplement. However, you should never use raw eggs, due to the risk of getting salmonella.

### Double strength milk recipe:

- Blend 1-cup dry skim milk powder into 1-quart milk.

You can buy protein supplements at drug stores and health food stores. They are available as powder that can be mixed with liquids or foods.

### If you are lactose intolerant

Low lactose milks (Lactaid©), cheeses and ice cream are available. People who are mildly lactose intolerant can often tolerate yogurt and fattier dairy foods such as cheese and ice cream. Soymilk, almond milk, coconut milk and rice milk, which are non-dairy products, can be substituted for milk. Lactaid© pills, which contain the enzyme that digests milk, can be taken before eating dairy foods. They are available at most drug stores.

# FLUID

## The Importance of Hydration

Dehydration occurs when a person does not take in enough fluid or loses too much fluid. Without enough water, the human body cannot function properly. In particular, people undergoing chemotherapy may be at a higher risk for dehydration due to treatment side effects, such as diarrhea and vomiting. Learning how to stay hydrated and recognizing and treating dehydration before it becomes severe are important steps for good health.

## Water and the body

Two-thirds of the human body is made up of water. Although it is possible to go for a long time without food, people cannot live without water for more than a few days. Every cell and organ depends on water to perform essential functions. The water in your body performs the following functions:

- Removes waste and toxins
- Transports nutrients and oxygen
- Controls heart rate and blood pressure
- Regulates body temperature
- Lubricates joints
- Protects organs and tissue, including the eyes, ears, and heart
- Creates saliva

## Causes of dehydration

The average adult loses more than 10 cups of water every day through natural body functions, such as breathing, sweating, and going to the bathroom. Most people easily replace that fluid through drinking and eating. However, certain conditions affect the body's ability to stay well hydrated, requiring a conscious effort to take in more water. In fact, thirst is not a sufficient measure because a person may be dehydrated and not feel thirsty. Causes of dehydration include the following:

**Diarrhea, nausea, and vomiting.** People undergoing cancer treatments, such as chemotherapy, may experience these symptoms, which increase dehydration risk.

**Fever.** A high fever can result in dehydration. Patients undergoing cancer treatment may be at risk for infections, and a fever is usually a sign of infection.

**Age.** Infants, children, and older adults are at greater risk for dehydration. Although young children don't weigh much, they pass water and electrolytes (minerals that help regulate the body) out of the body frequently. They also are likely to get diarrhea, a common childhood illness. Meanwhile, as a person gets older, the body slowly loses the ability to conserve water. Older adults are also at risk because they are less likely to sense that they are thirsty and may not eat or drink enough, especially if they live alone. Illnesses, disabilities, and certain medications can also contribute to dehydration.

**Other chronic illness.** Many diseases, such as diabetes, cystic fibrosis (a disease in which thick mucus affects the lungs and digestive system), and kidney disease, increase dehydration risk and/or need for fluids. For example, people with uncontrolled diabetes urinate frequently. Also, some medications can cause a person to urinate or sweat more than normal.

**Environment.** Living, working, and exercising in a hot or humid environment increase the need for fluids. People living at high altitudes (from 8,000 feet to 12,000 feet) also need more fluids because their bodies lose water as they work to take in more oxygen.

**Exercise.** Everyone loses water through sweat, and people who engage in physical activity generally produce a significant amount of sweat. Even if you don't see sweat, you are likely sweating. The more you exercise the more fluid replacement you need.

**Other factors.** Women and overweight or obese individuals are at greater risk for dehydration.

## Dehydration symptoms

Dehydration is cumulative, meaning the longer you go without enough fluids, the more dehydrated you will become. Although thirst is one way your body alerts you to drink more, other symptoms of dehydration include the following:

- A dry or sticky mouth or a swollen tongue
- Fatigue, weakness
- Irritability
- Dizziness, lightheadedness
- Nausea
- Headaches
- Constipation
- Dry skin
- Weight loss
- Dark yellow urine or a decrease in urination

Severe dehydration, which can be life-threatening and needs immediate medical treatment, can cause the following symptoms:

- Extreme thirst
- Fever
- Rapid heartbeat
- Lack of urination for more than eight hours
- Sunken eyes
- Inability to sweat
- Inability to produce tears
- Low blood pressure
- Disorientation or confusion

**Drink adequate fluids.** Drinking at least eight cups of water each day is a good rule of thumb, according to the Academy of Nutrition Dietetics. However, if you have any risk factors for dehydration, you should drink more. If you dislike plain water, try drinking a flavored water or adding a slice of lemon. Other fluids, such as juice and tea, contribute to your fluid count, as well.

**Eat foods with high water content.** While drinking water is the best source of hydration, many foods contain water and can help replenish lost fluids. Choose foods like lettuce (95% water), watermelon (92% water), and broccoli (91% water). Soups, popsicles, and yogurt also have high water content.

**Get help managing side effects.** If you are undergoing a treatment, such as chemotherapy, that is causing nausea, vomiting, or diarrhea, talk with your clinical team about ways to prevent or minimize these side effects.

**Don't wait to drink.** Make a conscious effort to drink enough on a regular basis and more often when you begin feeling ill, before you exercise, or before you go out into hot weather. Ensuring that you are well hydrated before you lose water can help reduce your risk for dehydration.

**Avoid foods and drinks that may contribute to dehydration.** Beverages with sugar and/ or caffeine (such as fruit juice, soda, and coffee) may help to hydrate some, but they are not as effective as low-sugar or low/non-caffeine beverages.

## Treating dehydration

If you are experiencing side effects from cancer treatment or an illness and find it hard to take in and keep down water and food, it can be difficult to replace the water your body has lost. Try these tips to address mild dehydration:

- Suck on ice chips or popsicles if you are having trouble drinking water or eating.
- Apply moisturizer to cracked lips and medication to mouth sores so that drinking and eating is less painful.

- If you are able to drink, take in small amounts frequently instead of a large amount at one time; drinking too much fluid at once may cause vomiting.
- Keep a water bottle with you at all times, and sip throughout the waking hours.
- Drink a large glass of water before bed and when you awake each morning.
- If you have diarrhea, be sure to select beverages that have sodium and potassium to help replace these losses in stool.
- If you have fatigue, keep ice and drinks within reach so you don't have to get up more often than necessary.

## What is dehydration?

Dehydration is an excessive loss of body fluids. It occurs when the output of fluid exceeds fluid intake.

- Side effects of treatment such as vomiting or diarrhea can lead to chemotherapy dehydration.
- Infections, high fever, bleeding, or even something as simple as not drinking enough fluids can also lead to dehydration.
- The danger of dehydration is greatest for a person living alone, as he/she may not recognize the signs and effects of dehydration.
- *Chemotherapy Dehydration* is a dangerous symptom, one that can be life threatening if the signs are not recognized and treated. When a person suffers from dehydrated, he may need to seek medical help to receive intravenous fluids. A person can live for a long time without eating, but can function only a short time without fluids.
- Electrolytes, such as potassium and sodium, are always present in the blood. When these electrolytes are too high or too low, they can cause problems. Some can be life-threatening. Confusion and disorientation are symptoms of dehydration resulting from an electrolyte imbalance. Thus, a person who is having severe vomiting or diarrhea should not be left alone to care for him or herself. When a person suffers from dehydration, it is difficult to judge how well he/she is doing and whether or not he/she needs help because of this confusion.

### What are some dehydration symptoms to look for?

- Dry mucous membranes (dry mouth)
- Your skin may appear loose and crinkled and could keep standing up in a tent when lightly pinched and pulled up.
- Secretions may become thick and dry.
- Little or no urine output.

### Things you can do to manage the effects of dehydration:

- **The best way to treat chemotherapy dehydration is to prevent it.** Recognize early symptoms of dehydration such as thirst and dry mouth and take steps to rehydrate yourself. Try to estimate how much fluid is lost and how much is taken in. It is not easy to tell how much fluid a person is losing unless it is being measured. Keeping a count of how many times a person is having diarrhea or vomiting may be easier than actually measuring the amount, and this information will be very helpful when talking to the doctor about chemotherapy dehydration symptoms. It is also important to keep track of how much fluid is taken in.

- **Increase fluid intake**. If fluids cannot be kept down, sometimes taking small pieces of ice works better, but it takes a lot of ice to get enough fluid. Taking small sips frequently is better tolerated than drinking large amounts. Fluids such as water, soda, bouillon, juice, or whatever is tolerated can be tried. Alcohol and caffeine should be avoided because they increase the effects of dehydration.
- **Minimize or eliminate fluid loss when signs of dehydration are present**. The first step is to stop the diarrhea or vomiting and to continue drinking fluids to replace those lost. Stopping diarrhea or vomiting usually requires medication. If pills are vomited, rectal suppositories are available. In some cases of chemotherapy dehydration, an injection may be needed.

## Vomiting

- If you are vomiting, stop eating. Once you stop vomiting, start back on food slowly. Start with small amounts of clear liquids, such as broth, juice soda, sports drinks, or water. Then, advance to light, mild foods like gelatin, bananas, rice, or toast. If you are not back to solid foods within a day or two, seek medical attention.
- Avoid caffeine and smoking when symptoms of dehydration are present.
- Suck on hard candy, popsicles, or ice if you are susceptible to chemotherapy dehydration.
- Take the medications for nausea and vomiting as prescribed by your doctor. If you are running low, ask for a refill.
- Notify your medical team if you feel nauseated during chemotherapy.

## Taste Changes

The most common oral side effects of outpatient chemotherapy are altered taste sensation (52%), dry mouth (35%) and mucositis (22%). All these side effects are unpleasant and may have a significant effect on a patient's quality of life. (40) The main reason your taste of food changes has to do with the nature of chemo therapy itself. The purpose is to attack cancer cells which grow rapidly. Drugs most commonly associated with taste changes include carboplatin, cisplatin, cyclophosphamide, dacarbazine, dactinomycin, doxorubicin, 5-fluorouracil, levamisole, mechlorethamine, methotrexate, paclitaxel, and vincristine. Most people report taste changes involving a lower threshold for bitter tastes and a higher threshold for sweet tastes. Some drugs also produce a metal taste during the actual intravenous infusion. These include nitrogen mustard, vincristine, cisplatin, and cyclophosphamide. Taste changes may occur during therapy and last for hours, days, weeks, or even months after chemotherapy.

## Management

Notify your medical team if you are suffering from taste changes to come up with a tailored individualized plan, suitable for your medical needs.

Using spices like cumin, cinnamon, coriander. If tasting metal, add acid like citrus found in lemons, limes and oranges. If you feel like you are eating cardboard, add salt. Sea salt is best because it's not processed like typical table salt. If foods taste bitter or harsh try drops of Grade B organic maple or honey.

Fat is encouraged and recognized a natural flavor carrier. It is suggested to eat healthy fats like olive oil, nuts, avocado, and coconut oil. "Fat is like a magic carpet traversing back and forth across your palate, delivering tastes," she says, "so all of a sudden you have that involuntary spasm of vocal delight, turning yuck into yum." (29)

Several studies have looked at the use of zinc sulfate in mitigating taste alterations, but conflicting findings have resulted. Some found that zinc supplementation increased recovery in taste acuity, but some found that zinc supplementation had no effect on taste alteration. (41, 42, 43). This treatment should be used with caution until further research confirms its efficacy because excessive zinc supplementation can negatively impact the immune system. (44).

## Supplements

Supplements are vitamins and minerals, herbal remedies, protein powders, and shakes that are designed and intended to supply nutrients when you are not able to meet your needs through diet alone.

In an ideal world we should be able to gather all our vitamins and nutrients from food sources. However some people are not acquiring them secondary to poor dietary habits and also the requirements change based on specific medical conditions. With all these in mind it is advisable to use vitamins and supplements that will help your body maintain an optimal function.

The length of time that you are on a supplement mostly depends on the intention; if it is being given to support health in general you might need certain supplements to be taken continuously such as multivitamins, Vitamin D and Calcium, along with shakes and smoothies. However if you are taking it during a specific time in your life or for specific conditions it might only be required during a short period of time as in the case of some protein powders and supplemental shakes. Your health care provider, dietitian, and medical team can help you make the correct decision.

## Sugar

The thought that sugar feeds cancer is a current topic. To cut to the chase: it's not that simple. There is not a 1:1 ratio or direct link between eating a bite of sugar and the resulting growth of a certain number of cancer cells. "Sugar" is a term often used to represent dozens of important, natural chemical structures that exist in our bodies. However, most of us hear the word sugar and visualize the white form of table sugar.

The typical American diet is high in many processed and refined foods, including sugar and white flour. Replacing these foods with healthy forms of carbohydrates, such as fruits and whole grains, is advised for people who have had cancer. However, being fearful of or restricting intake of certain foods that contain natural sugars is not necessary or healthful.

Here's an example: Should cancer survivors avoid eating fruits because they have natural sugar? For comparison's sake, let's consider that one medium orange contains 12 grams of sugar and a small donut contains 10 grams of sugar. The difference is that the orange also contains fiber and phytonutrients, both of which may play a role in fighting cancer, whereas the donut is just 200 empty calories, devoid of any potential nutritional benefit. Eliminating foods that contain sugar, such as fruits, is not wise for cancer survivors as this limits intake of cancer-fighting nutrients that are important for energy and overall health.

In fact, many cancer patients are led to believe they must follow a restricted sugar diet for fear of causing cancer growth in themselves if they do not adhere. This fear and rigidity often promotes a very stressful experience. The stress will actually lead to an increase in blood sugar as well as compromised immunity. These negative health effects are actually the exact opposite of the purported benefit of such a plan.

There may be a connection, however, between a diet high in refined, processed foods combined with a sedentary lifestyle that may lead a person to become overweight and eventually experience insulin resistance. Insulin resistance can cause an increase in blood levels of insulin and related compounds that may act as growth factors. The connection between body weight, insulin levels and cancer survivorship is currently being researched. In the meantime, becoming more physically active, striving to maintain a healthy weight and eating a plant-based diet including substituting refined sugars and white flour with whole grains and other unprocessed carbohydrates can all help to keep insulin levels in check and promote cancer survivorship.

## Prepare Yourself

1) **Optimize your weight:** If you have lost weight, seek ways to obtain more calories, protein and fluid. Ask to speak a registered dietitian working with your team to make a tailored meal plan by using an eating strategy prior to entering into your chemotherapy regimen.

2) **Bring nourishments:** If you know you are going to be out for the day, and/or at a chemotherapy session for more than 2 hours, be sure to bring a "high-protein snacks" (*refer to list*), fluids, and/or a meal.

3) **Obtain Support:** If you need help for food, shopping, meal preparation be sure to speak to your medical team about support. If you don't have family or friends to help with this, you will want to address these needs with a social worker and a registered dietitian that works with you team.

4) **Increase your good fat levels:** We have known for a while about the positive benefits of omega 3 in the cancer process. Fish oils provide the long-chain version, which helps to reduce cellular inflammation. Short-chain omega 3 can be found in flaxseeds and walnuts. Organic olive oil has major benefits in the intestine and can displace bad fats in the body.

5) **Attend Support classes**: Knowledge is key. Increasing your mental expectations and gaining insight on experiences can be helpful. It can also be helpful to create supportive connections, such as meeting clinical staff members and other patient survivors. If your chemotherapy center does not offer support classes your local library or health store may.

6) **Exercise**: You should exercise, even the least strenuous forms of yoga. It will add oxygen into your blood by getting you to breathe better and it will reduce levels of toxins in the body and rebalance hormones. It is understandable that for some people on chemotherapy this is just impossible. The simple fact is that research shows that light daily exercise of about 30 minutes duration helps improve survival rates by up to 50 per cent.

7) **Be aware of possible diet alterations while on chemotherapy**: Sometimes special "diets" are used to maximize tolerance and avoid chemotherapy complications related to the diet. A registered dietitian working with your medical team can help determine the best diet and meal plan for you. The diets may include:

- **Clear Liquid** This diet includes fruit juice, gelatin, popsicles, broth, fruit ice, coffee, and tea. It is usually for after surgery awaiting digestion to return, as well as for bowel rest with vomiting and diarrhea.
- **Full Liquid** This diet includes milk, yogurt without fruit pieces, ice cream, sherbet, milkshakes, strained cream soups, hot cereal, commercial supplements, custard and pudding. It is intended as a progression from clear liquids or for individuals who have difficulty swallowing solid foods due to a narrowed esophagus or mouth or throat pain.
- **Soft/Low Fiber** A soft diet avoids raw fruits and vegetables, and foods that have skins, nuts, seeds, etc. It may be indicated for patients at moderate risk for a bowel obstruction (blockage), which may be a result of pain or anti-nausea medications causing extreme constipation. A low fiber diet omits all fruit and vegetables except fruit juice and white potatoes. It also avoids most foods containing fiber such as grains. This diet is meant only for patients whose bowel may be partially obstructed or are at very high risk for an obstruction.

- **Low Lactose** A low lactose diet avoids foods that contain lactose, a naturally occurring milk sugar. This diet is appropriate for patients who are lactose intolerant or experience gas, bloating, cramping, or diarrhea after eating products that contain lactose. It also may be necessary to follow a low lactose diet if these types of symptoms develop related to cancer treatments.
- **High Calorie / High Protein** In order to maintain your weight before, during, or after treatments you may need to eat foods or beverages that are high in calories and protein. It may be necessary to add calorie boosters to your foods or beverages or include protein supplements. This can help you avoid or minimize weight loss and maximize energy and strength.
- **Carbohydrate Controlled** A carbohydrate controlled diet may be used for patients who experience medication related hyperglycemia or blood sugar spikes. This diet focuses on controlling servings of carbohydrate containing foods such as grains, starchy vegetables, fruits and dairy products. Meals and snacks are mixed to include protein and nutritious fats in addition to carbohydrates.
- **Neutropenic** A neutropenic diet is a low bacteria diet. This may be used for patients whose cancer treatment alters infection-fighting White Blood Cells called Neutrophils. Some of these foods include raw and unpasteurized foods that may make you susceptible to an infection if you have neutrophils.

Your cancer is as individual as you are, so your treatment package needs to be tailored specifically to you and your cancer. At least half of all cancers are caused by poor lifestyle. Other cancers may be caused by environmental toxins or other reasons. Cancer can take many years to develop, so be patient, do your best to be and feel your best.

- When eating to meet your daily five a day of colorful plant foods, think of a Rainbow (46). Think rainbow or ROY-G-BIV (an acronym for remembering the colors of the rainbow). Yes, red, orange, yellow, green, blue, indigo and violet are colors you want to eat daily.

R-RED        O-Orange        Y-Yellow        G-Green        B-Blue        I-Indigo        V-Violet

**AICR Phytochemicals**

| Phytochemical(s) | Plant Source | Possible Benefits |
|---|---|---|
| Carotenoids (such as beta-carotene, lycopene, lutein, zeaxanthin) | Red, orange and green fruits and vegetables including broccoli, carrots, cooked tomatoes, leafy greens, sweet potatoes, winter squash, apricots, cantaloupe, oranges and watermelon | May inhibit cancer cell growth, work as antioxidants and improve immune response |
| Flavonoids (such as anthocyanins and quercetin) | Apples, citrus fruits, onions, soybeans and soy products (tofu, soy milk, edamame, etc.), coffee and tea | May inhibit inflammation and tumor growth; may aid immunity and boost production of detoxifying enzymes in the body |
| Indoles and Glucosinolates (sulforaphane) | Cruciferous vegetables (broccoli, cabbage, collard greens, kale, cauliflower and Brussels sprouts) | May induce detoxification of carcinogens, limit production of cancer-related hormones, block carcinogens and prevent tumor growth |

| Phytochemical(s) | Plant Source | Possible Benefits |
|---|---|---|
| Inositol (phytic acid) | Bran from corn, oats, rice, rye and wheat, nuts, soybeans and soy products (tofu, soy milk, edamame, etc.) | May retard cell growth and work as antioxidant |
| Isoflavones (daidzein and genistein) | Soybeans and soy products (tofu, soy milk, edamame, etc.) | May inhibit tumor growth, limit production of cancer-related hormones and generally work as antioxidant |
| Isothiocyanates | Cruciferous vegetables (broccoli, cabbage, collard greens, kale, cauliflower and Brussels sprouts) | May induce detoxification of carcinogens, block tumor growth and work as antioxidants |
| Polyphenols (such as ellagic acid and resveratrol) | Green tea, grapes, wine, berries, citrus fruits, apples, whole grains and peanuts | May prevent cancer formation, prevent inflammation and work as antioxidants |
| Terpenes (such as perillyl alcohol, limonene, carnosol) | Cherries, citrus fruit peel, rosemary | May protect cells from becoming cancerous, slow cancer cell growth, strengthen immune function, limit production of cancer-related hormones, fight viruses, work as antioxidants |

## Sample Menus (47)

*Menu 1.*

*Breakfast 1 serving whole-grain cereal with berries, fat-free or lowfat milk or yogurt, 6 oz. orange juice*

*Lunch 5-minute microwave-baked sweet potato, steamed broccoli, 1 Tablespoons salsa, 1 oz. cheddar cheese, 1 apple or other piece of fruit*

*Dinner 1 serving Oven Roasted Fish Mediterranean Style\*, ¼ cantaloupe topped with ½ cup fresh or frozen and thawed strawberries*

*Menu 2.*

*Breakfast 2 Tablespoons low-fat cottage or ricotta cheese and 1 tsp. all-fruit preserves spread on 8-inch whole-wheat tortilla and rolled up, 6 oz. reduced-sodium vegetable juice*

*Lunch Romaine, tomato and chickpea salad\* with quartered hard-boiled egg, lite vinaigrette dressing, 1 slice whole-grain bread, 1 cup red grapes*

*Dinner 1 cup minestrone soup, 1 serving Veggie-Turkey Loaf\*, 1 small whole-grain roll, steamed broccoli drizzled with olive oil, ½ cup mango sorbet with ½ cup mixed berries (frozen and thawed if fresh are not in season)*

**Menu 3**.

*Breakfast 1 whole-grain mini bagel (or half regular size bagel), 2 oz. canned and drained salmon mixed with 1 oz. low-fat cream cheese or Neufchatel cheese, slice of honeydew melon*

*Lunch 1 large whole-wheat pita bread with 2 tablespoons hummus, grated carrot, sliced tomato and zucchini and green pepper strips, 1 cup cherries (frozen and thawed if fresh are not in season)*

*Dinner 3 oz. herb-roasted skinless chicken breast\*, 1 serving Cider-Glazed Sweet Potatoes with Cranberries, steamed baby Brussels sprouts, 1 fresh pear or 1 cup pears canned in juice*

**Menu 4**.

*Breakfast 2 eggs scrambled in 1 tsp. canola oil in nonstick pan, 2 slices whole-grain toast with all-fruit preserves, ½ grapefruit*

*Lunch 1 serving Boston Bean Soup\*, 3 low-fat whole-grain crackers made with 0 trans-fat, raw vegetables (cauliflower, red pepper, celery and carrots) with salsa dip, 1 cup fresh blueberries (or frozen and thawed)*

*Dinner 1 serving Penne and Tuna\*, red leaf lettuce salad with artichoke hearts, red onion and mushrooms, iced tea, 1 seasonal fruit (peach, pear, or kiwi)*

**Menu 5**.

*Breakfast 1 cup oatmeal with raisins and cinnamon, topped with chopped apple, 6 oz. orange juice, ½ cup vanilla low-fat yogurt*

*Lunch 3 oz. meatloaf\* sandwich on whole-wheat bread with mustard and sliced onion, garden salad with low-fat vinaigrette, 1 cup fresh fruit salad*

*Dinner 1 serving Classic Stir-Fry served over brown rice\* (included in recipe), ½ cup pineapple chunks canned in juice*

**Menu 6**.

*Breakfast 1 Tbsp. natural peanut butter on whole-grain bread with all-fruit preserves OR 6 oz. low-fat yogurt mixed with fresh*

*Lunch 3 oz. sliced white meat turkey\* on whole-grain bread with sliced tomato, 2 slices of avocado and sliced red onion, small slice angel cake topped with ½ cup raspberries (frozen and thawed if fresh not available)*

*Dinner 1 cup roasted zucchini, carrots, onion and asparagus lightly drizzled with balsamic vinegar\*, ½ cup cooked whole grains (try barley, bulgur, kasha or millet), 1 serving Apple and Pork Stir-Fry with Ginger\*.*

## Menu 7.

*Breakfast Small low-fat muffin, ½ cup low fat cottage cheese mixed with sprinkle dried fruit*

*Lunch 1 serving Easy Lentil Soup\*, whole-grain pita bread, green salad with watercress or endive and low-fat vinaigrette dressing, fresh fruit (1 cup chopped fruit, berries, or 1 whole apple or pear)*

*Dinner 1 serving Superbowl Chili Mac\*, 1 cup Cole slaw, ½ cup cherries (frozen then thawed) with ½ cup low-fat frozen vanilla yogurt*

*\*recipes found http://www.aicr.org/enews/archived/menus-for-the-new-american-plate.html*

1. Jennifer A. Ligibel, Catherine M. Alfano American Society of Clinical Oncology Position Statement on Obesity and Cancer.
2. http://www.cancer.gov/cancertopics/factsheet/risk/obesity.
3. Diaz ES[1], Karlan BY, Li AJ. Obesity-associated adipokines correlate with survival in epithelial ovarian cancer, Gynecol Oncol. 2013 May;129(2):353
4. Baldwin, C., Spiro, A., Ahern, R., & Emery, P. W. (2012). Oral nutritional interventions in malnourished patients with cancer: A systematic review and meta-analysis. *Journal of the National Cancer Institute*, *104*(5), 371-385.
5. Ilaria Ronga, Anorexia–cachexia syndrome in pancreatic cancer: Recent advances and new pharmacological approach. Advances in Medical Sciences Volume 59, Issue 1, March 2014, Pages 1–6
6. Hopkinson JB, MacDonald J, Wright DNM, Corner JL. The prevalence of concern about weight loss and change in eating habits in people with advanced cancer. J Pain Symptom Manag. 2006;32:322–331

Inui A. Cancer anorexia-cachexia syndrome: current issues in research and management. CA Cancer J Clin. 2002;52:72–91.

7. MacDonald N, Easson AM, Mazurak VC, et al. Understanding and managing cancer cachexia. J Am Coll Surg. 2003;197:143–61.
8. Evans WJ, Morley JE, Argiles J, et al. Cachexia: a new definition. Clin Nutr. 2008;27:793
9. Bamini Gopinath, Consumption of polyunsaturated fatty acids, fish, and nuts and risk of inflammatory disease mortality. American journal of Clinical Nutrition, 2011
10. Conlon, B. (2010). Malnutrition and malabsorptive diarrhea in pancreatic cancer. *Oncology Nutrition Connection*, *18*(4), 10-21.
11. Datema, F. R., Ferrier, M. B., & Baatenburg de Jong, R. J. (2011). Impact of severe malnutrition on short-term mortality and overall survival in head and neck cancer. *Oral Oncology*, *47*(9), 910-914.
12. Elia, M. (2011). Oral nutritional support in patients with cancer of the gastrointestinal tract. *Journal of Human Nutrition and Dietetics*, *24*(5), 417-420.
13. O'Mara, A., & St. Germain, D. (2012). Improved outcomes in the malnourished patient: We're not there yet. *Journal of the National Cancer Institute*, *104*(5), 342-343.
14. Pepersack, T. (2011). For an operational definition of cachexia. *Lancet Oncology*, *12*(5), 423-424.

15. Rebar, C. R., & Ignatavicius, D. D. (2013). Care of patients with malnutrition and obesity. In D. D. Ignatavicius, & M. L. Workman (Eds.), *Medical surgical nursing: Patient-centered collaborative care* (7th ed., pp. 1340-1349). St. Louis: Elsevier Saunders.

16. Schulmeister, L. (2007). Nutrition. In M. E. Langhorne, J. S. Fulton, & S. E. Otto (Eds.), *Oncology nursing* (5th ed., pp. 465-475). St. Louis: Mosby Elsevier.

17. Ashrafian H, Ahmed K, Rowland SP, et al. Metabolic surgery and cancer: protective effects of bariatric procedures. *Cancer* 2011; 117(9):1788–1799.

18. Ballard-Barbash R, Berrigan D, Potischman N, Dowling E. Obesity and cancer epidemiology. In: Berger NA, editor. *Cancer and Energy Balance, Epidemiology and Overview.* New York: Springer-Verlag New York, LLC, 2010.

19. Ballard-Barbash R, Hunsberger S, Alciati MH. Physical activity, weight control, and breast cancer risk and survival: clinical trial rationale and design considerations. *Journal of the National Cancer Institute* 2009; 101(9):630–643.

20. Flegal KM, Carroll MD, Ogden CL, Curtin LR. Prevalence and trends in obesity among US adults, 1999–2008. *JAMA* 2010; 303(3):235–241.

21. Grivennikov SI, Greten FR, Karin M. Immunity, inflammation, and cancer. *Cell* 2010; 140(6):883–899.

22. National Heart, Lung, and Blood Institute (1998). *Clinical Guidelines on the Identification, Evaluation, and Treatment of Overweight and Obesity in Adults: The Evidence Report.* NIH Publication No. 98–4083. Bethesda, MD.

23. Ogden CL, Carroll MD, Curtin LR, Lamb MM, Flegal KM. Prevalence of high body mass index in US children and adolescents, 2007–2008. *JAMA* 2010; 303(3):242–249.

24. Polednak AP. Estimating the number of U.S. incident cancers attributable to obesity and the impact on temporal trends in incidence rates for obesity-related cancers. *Cancer Detection and Prevention* 2008; 32(3):190–199.

25. Roberts DL, Dive C, Renehan AG. Biological mechanisms linking obesity and cancer risk: new perspectives. *Annual Review of Medicine* 2010; 61:301–316.

26. Wang YC, McPherson K, Marsh T, Gortmaker SL, Brown M. Health and economic burden of the projected obesity trends in the USA and the UK. *Lancet* 2011; 378(9793):815–825

27. Wolin KY, Carson K, Colditz GA. Obesity and cancer. *Oncologist* 2010; 15(6):556–565

28. Katrina VB. Claghorn, M.S., R.D., L.D.N. Protein needs during cancer treatment. Oncolink - Cancer.2012 *www.oncolink.org/coping/article*

29. http://www.npr.org/2014/04/07/295800503/chemo-can-make-food-taste-like-metal-heres-help

30. http://www.cancerresearchuk.org/about-cancer/cancers-in-general/treatment/cancer-drugs/megestrol

31. Christopher T. Hensley*J Glutamine and cancer: cell biology, physiology, and clinical opportunities Clin Invest.* 2013;123(9):3678–3684

32. Kuhn KS[1], Muscaritoli M, Wischmeyer P, Stehle P. Glutamine as indispensable nutrient in oncology: experimental and clinical evidence. Eur J Nutr. 2010 Jun;49(4):197-210. doi: 10.1007/s00394-009-0082-2. Epub 2009 Nov

33. Lawenda, Brian, *Use Glutamine To Reduce The Severity Of Mucositis And Neuropathy (During Chemotherapy Or Radiation Therapy,* February 25, 2013

34. Motallebnejad M[1], Akram S, Moghadamnia A, Moulana Z, Omidi S., J Contemp Dent Pract. *The effect of topical application of pure honey on radiation-induced mucositis: a randomized clinical trial.* 2008 Mar 1;9(3):40-7.

35. Maiti PK[1,] Ray A, Mitra TN, Jana U, Bhattacharya J, Ganguly SJ Indian Med Assoc *The effect of honey on mucositis induced by chemo-radiation in head and neck cancer..*2012 Jul;110(7):453-6. Chin J Integr Med. 2012 Aug;18(8):635-40. doi: 10.1007/s11655-012-1183-y. Epub 2012 Aug 2.

36. *Greg Arnold,* Potential prevention: Aloe vera mouthwash may reduce radiation-induced oral mucositis in head and neck cancer patients. *January 17, 2013*

37. Oral mucositis due to cancer treatments. Orodental hygiene and ice cubes. Prescrire Int. 2008 Feb;17(93):33-5.

38. Flavia, Castelino and Elsa, Sanatombi Devi and Jyothi, RK (2011) *Effectiveness of Plain Ice Cubes Versus Flavoured Ice Cubes in Preventing Oral Mucositis associated with Injection 5-Fluorouracil among Cancer Patients.* International Journal of Nursing Education, 3 (2). pp. 38-40. ISSN 0974-9349

39. Wilson J[1], Rees JS, The dental treatment needs and oral side effects of patients undergoing outpatient cancer chemotherapy. Eur J Prosthodont Restor Dent. 2005 Sep;13(3):129-34.

40. Ripamonti, C., Zecca, E., Brunelli, C., Fulfaro, F., Villa, S., Balzarini, A.,...Conno, F. (1998). A randomized, controlled clinical trial to evaluate the effects of zinc sulfate on cancer patients with taste alterations caused by head and neck irradiation. *Cancer, 82,* 1938-1945

41. Yamagata, T., Nakamura, Y., Yamagata, Y., Nakanishi, M., Matsunaga, K., Nakanishi, H., Yukawa, S. (2003). The pilot trial of the prevention of the increase in electrical taste thresholds by zinc containing fluid infusion during chemotherapy to treat primary lung cancer. *Journal of Experimental and Clinical Cancer Research, 22,* 557-63.

42. Halyard, M. Y., Jatoi, A., Sloan, J. A., Bearden, J. D., Vora, S. A., Atherton, P. J., Loprinzi, C. L. (2007). Does zinc sulfate prevent therapy-induced taste alterations in head and neck cancer patients, Results of phase III double-blind, placebo-controlled trial from the north central cancer treatment group (N01C4). *International Journal of Radiation Oncology, Biology, Physics, 67,* 13-18-1322.

43. Peregrin, T. (2006). Improving taste sensation in patients who have undergone chemotherapy or radiation therapy. *Journal of the American Dietetic Association, 106,* 1536-1540

44. Nathaniel J. Szewczyk, Lewis A. Jacobson. Signal-transduction networks and the regulation of muscle protein degradation. The International Journal of Biochemistry & Cell Biology Volume 37, Issue 10, October 2005, Pages 1997–2011

45. www.**aicr**.org/new-american-plate/nap-challenge/week-9.html

46. http://www.aicr.org/enews/archived/menus-for-the-new-american-plate.html

Printed in the United States
By Bookmasters